THE HERBAL COOKBOOK

Using Nature's Pharmacy in the Kitchen

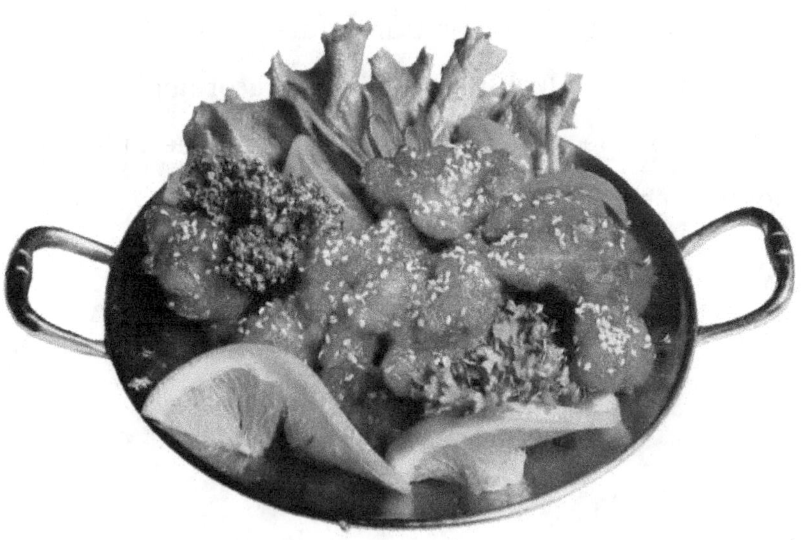

JONATHAN O. KELVIN

COPYRIGHT © 2024

All rights reserved. Except for brief quotations included in critical reviews and certain other noncommercial uses allowed by copyright law, no part of this publication may be reproduced, distributed, or transmitted in any form or by any means, including photocopying, recording, or other electronic or mechanical methods, without the publisher's prior written permission.

ACKNOWLEDGEMENT

I sincerely thank everyone whose assistance and contributions made this book possible. With sincere gratitude, I would like to thank [my family, friends and wellwishers] for their constant support, direction, and encouragement during this journey. I owe them for their knowledge, commitment, and inspiration

TABLE OF CONTENTS

INTRODUCTION

Welcome to "The Herbal Cookbook: Using Nature's Pharmacy in the Kitchen," where the fascinating world of herbs and spices collides with the skill of culinary alchemy. This cookbook is an ode to the abundant pharmacy of nature, bringing the seductive charm of herbs into your kitchen and turning cooking into a savory and aromatic adventure.

We set off on a gastronomic journey in this entrancing compilation that skillfully combines the delights of cooking with the ancient knowledge of herbalism. Imagine your kitchen as a sanctuary where the fragrances of rosemary, thyme, and basil fill the air, enhancing the flavor and healthfulness of every meal. The Herbal Cookbook is more than simply a list of recipes; it's a call to investigate the symbiotic link between food and plants, which improves health and flavor.

Enter a realm where the rich tapestry of herbal cuisine is revealed with each turn of the page. This cookbook is a veritable gold mine of mouthwatering options, ranging from garden-fresh treats to fusion masterpieces with global inspiration. Find out how adding even the most basic herbs to your cooking can raise even the most conventional dishes into remarkable experiences.

Beyond the delicious flavors, these dishes use herbs' inherent therapeutic qualities to turn your kitchen into a health haven. We explore the therapeutic uses of herbs, revealing how they may improve the flavor and nutritional value of your food. Use this cookbook as a guide to embrace the culinary potential of herbs in your everyday endeavors.

So come along on this fragrant adventure through "The Herbal Cookbook," regardless of your level of culinary experience. Allow the enchantment of herbs to stoke your love of cooking and reveal the astounding potential that nature's medicine has to offer your kitchen. Prepare to immerse yourself in a gastronomic journey that satisfies the senses and uplifts the spirit by adding the essence of herbs to your meals.

CHAPTER 1

Herbal Treats for Particular Events

In the chapter "Herbal Delights for Special Occasions" of "The Herbal Cookbook: Using Nature's Pharmacy in the Kitchen," you are invited to embark on a culinary adventure where the unadulterated essence of herbs takes your festivities to new directions. Herbal magic provides a touch of elegance and taste to your foods that capture the senses, whether you're hosting a joyful gathering, a family reunion, or an intimate dinner party.

1. Cocktails with Herb Infusions:
Inject your special occasion with a herbal freshness burst into your drink creations. Imagine something as visually lovely as a Lavender Lemonade Spritz or a Basil Berry Bliss, but much more delicious. Your guests will have a one-of-a-kind and unforgettable experience thanks to these herbal mixtures.

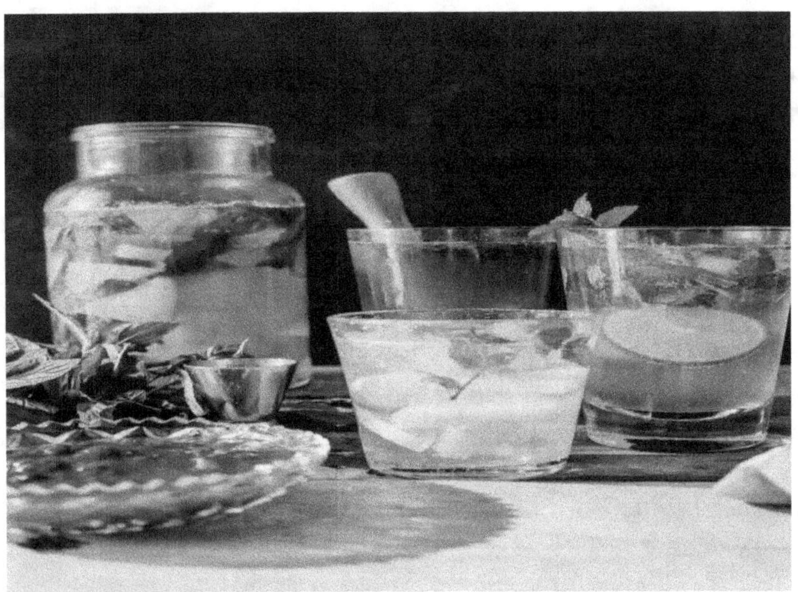

Recipe Example: Spritz of Lavender Lemonade
Ingredients: 1/4 cup lemon juice, fresh
Half a cup simple syrup flavored with lavender
sparkling water
Ice cubes Garnish with sprigs of lavender

2. Rosemary Roasted Lamb: This dish is a magnificent focal point that is sure to turn heads. The flavor of the meat is enhanced by the fragrant properties of the rosemary, transforming an ordinary dish into a masterpiece of cooking. This herbaceous delicacy, which highlights the flavorful combination of herbs and meat, is ideal for celebratory events.
A Sample Recipe for Roasted Lamb with Rosemary

Ingredients: Lamb leg
pristine rosemary
cloves of garlic
Olive oil
Add pepper and salt.

3. Minty Chocolate Indulgence: A minty chocolate indulgence adds a cool edge to desserts, which are the delicious culmination of every celebration. Chocolate and mint come together to provide a decadent treat that is sure to please. This dish is a lovely symphony of tastes, in addition to being visually pleasing.
One such recipe is for mint chocolate mousse.
Chocolate that is dark in color
mint leaves that are fresh
cream of whipping
Eggs and Sugar

4. Herbal Elegance in Plating: Use herbal elegance in plating to improve the foods' aesthetic appeal. To add a splash of color to salads or desserts, use edible flowers like pansies or nasturtiums. For a refined touch, top creamy soups with chopped dill or chives. Your meals' aesthetic attractiveness adds to the whole sensory experience.
A Sample of a Presentation Salad of Edible Flowers
Components:
mixed greens for salad
Flowers that are edible (nasturtiums, pansies)
Balsamic salad dressing

5. Sorbet with Basil Infused: A delicious option is a Basil Infused Sorbet, which may be enjoyed as a palette cleanser between meals or as a refreshing finish. This frozen delicacy gains an unexpected and energizing aspect from the pungent fragrance of basil. It's the ideal method for clearing and resetting the palate in preparation for the next dish.
Example Recipe: Fresh basil leaves; fresh basil infused sorbet
Water, sugar, and lemon juice

6. Matching Herbal Teas: Offer a well chosen assortment of herbal teas to go with your particular event. Provide a range that complements the tastes of your food. A mint-infused tea revives the taste after a filling main meal, while a calming chamomile tea pairs well with sweets.
Ingredients: chamomile tea bags; example pairing: chamomile honey tea
Slices of lemon honey

7. Thyme-Infused Cheese dish: Use thyme-infused ingredients to create an elegant cheese dish. A variety of artisanal cheeses, honey infused with thyme, and infused goat cheese offer a rich and varied experience. A traditional appetizer becomes a gourmet experience with the addition of herbs.
Example of a Platter: Cheese Selection with Thyme Infusion
Different cheeses
honey laced with thyme
Bread and crackers

8. Lemon Lavender Sorbet: Think about presenting Lavender Lemon Sorbet as a palate-cleansing treat. A sorbet that is elegant and delicious is made when the zesty freshness of lemon and the gentle floral tones of lavender are mixed. It's the ideal option to clear the palate and get it ready for the next delicious dish.
Ingredients for an exemplary recipe: simple syrup scented with lavender; lavender-lemon juice
freshly squeezed lemon juice
Water

9. Chocolate Truffles with Herbal Infusion: Infuse your chocolate truffles with herbs to surprise and delight your visitors with a rich treat. Whether it's mint, rosemary, or lavender, these herb-infused treats give a traditional dessert a distinctive spin. These truffles would be a lovely, customized party favor.
Chocolate Truffles with Mint Syrup, for Example
Chocolate that is dark in color
mint leaves that are fresh
thick cream

10. Cocoa powder for covering :
Try the Sage and Cranberry Roast Chicken if you're looking for a chicken dish that blends the acidity of cranberries with the earthiness of sage. Because of the vivid colors of the cranberries and the fragrant scent of the sage, this meal is not only a culinary feast but also a work of artistic beauty.
Example of a Recipe: Roast Chicken with Sage and Cranberries;

Ingredients: Whole chicken
fresh leaves of sage
cranberries
Olive oil
Add pepper and salt.

11. Champagne Cocktails with Herb Infusion:
Champagne drinks laced with herbs will elevate your toasts.
These bubbly beverages, such the Thyme Citrus Sparkler or the
Rosemary Raspberry Fizz, provide a touch of refinement to any
occasion. The sparkling experience is enhanced by the aromatic
herbs, which turn each sip into a party unto itself.
Recipe Example: Rosemary Raspberry Fizz; Ingredients: Simple
syrup flavored with rosemary
ripe raspberries
Sparkling wine, or champagne

12. Grilled Shrimp Skewers with Dill and Lemon: Wow your
visitors with these fragrant and tasty shrimp skewers. The juicy
shrimp gains brightness and depth from the mix of lemon and
dill. These skewers are a great conversation starter at any special
occasion in addition to being a delicious appetizer.
Grilled Shrimp Skewers with Dill and Lemon, as an Example
Recipe
Components: Jumbo shrimp
new dill
Zest of lemons
Garlic with olive oil

13. Herbal Dessert Garnishes: Use herbal garnishes to add flair to your dessert display. Cakes, tarts, and other sweet delights might benefit from the finishing touches of fresh mint leaves, basil chiffonade, or lavender buds. The whole flavor profile is enhanced and the visual attractiveness is further enhanced by the herbal accents.
Slices of lemon tart with basil chiffonade as a garnish
A fresh salad of basil

14. Tarragon and Citrus Infused Salmon: Use this combination to make a main dish that will steal the show. The taste of the fish is enhanced by the zesty citrus overtones and the aromatic tarragon.

CHAPTER 2

Fusion of Global Herbs

A captivating tapestry of sensations and scents has emerged in the culinary world as a result of the blending of cuisines from all over the world. We explore the fascinating world of Global Herbal Fusion in "The Herbal Cookbook: Using Nature's Pharmacy in the Kitchen," where herbs from many cultures come together to produce foods that entice the senses and honor the great diversity of nature's wealth.

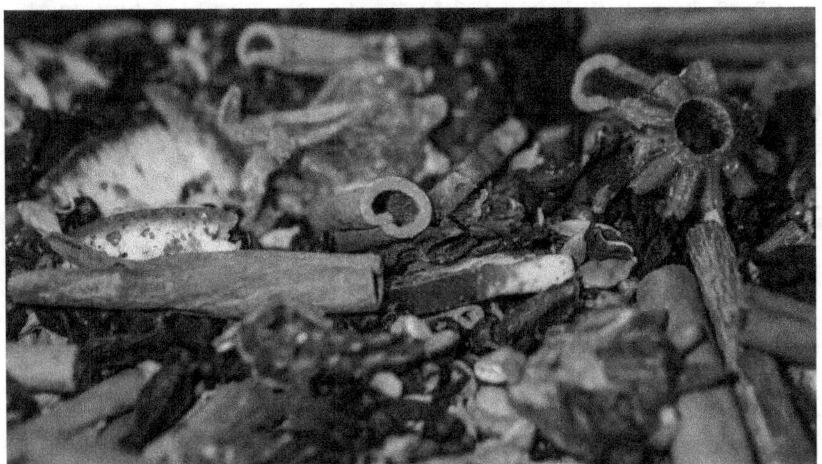

1. Comprehending the Fusion of Global Herbs: The technique of Global Herbal Fusion is combining herbs from many culinary traditions to produce meals that are distinctive and colorful. It's about discovering the complementing qualities of herbs from around the globe and dismantling barriers between cuisines.

2. Thai-Basil Infused Tacos: To make a fusion taco filling that combines the powerful tastes of Mexico with the freshness of Thai food, combine the fragrant Thai basil with Mexican seasonings. Every mouthful delivers a delightful rush of herbal deliciousness as a consequence.

3. Mediterranean Rosemary-Infused Pizza: Infuse the earthy scent of Mediterranean rosemary into the tomato sauce to elevate a traditional pizza. With each bite, this fusion cuisine captures the spirit of the Mediterranean, elevating the beloved classic Italian dish to new heights.

4. Indian-Italian Cilantro Pesto Pasta: This pasta recipe celebrates both cultures by combining the vibrant flavors of Indian cilantro with the classic Italian pesto sauce. The classic pesto made with basil is given a refreshing twist by the cilantro, which results in a symphony of tastes.

5. Sushi Rolls with a dash of Japanese Mint: Give your sushi rolls a light and fragrant twist by incorporating a dash of Japanese mint into them. This fusion gives the well-known meal a surprise herbal ingredient while embracing the delicate taste balance of Japanese cuisine.

6. Caribbean Jerk Chicken with Lemongrass Infusion: Infuse the traditional Caribbean jerk chicken with the zesty flavor of lemongrass. This is a unique culinary experience that combines ingredients that are spicy and lemony in a wonderful way.

7. French Lavender Crème Brûlée: Infuse the subtle lavender scent into the traditional French dessert, Crème Brûlée, to elevate it. This fusion dessert creates a very unforgettable delight by infusing a classic French pleasure with a hint of flowery elegance.

8. Greek Oregano-Infused Spanakopita: Infuse the filling with the fragrant fragrance of oregano to give the well-loved spinach pie a Greek touch. This fusion meal gives a nod to Greek tastes while updating a tried-and-true formula.

9. Mexican Cilantro-Lime Rice: Add the tangy taste of Mexican cilantro and lime to your rice meal to make it better. This fusion side dish gives a range of main meals the ideal balance of freshness and acidity.

The culinary innovation of "The Herbal Cookbook" is explored through Global Herbal Fusion, a concept in which herbs from across the world are combined to create recipes that cut over cultural barriers. We honor the beauty of herbs and the depth they provide to our kitchens by embracing the many flavors of various culinary traditions. These international herbal fusion recipes are perfect for home cooks or experienced chefs alike, as they take you on a worldwide culinary adventure inspired by the fragrant marvels of nature's pharmacy.

CHAPTER 3

Medicinal Appetizers

Take a culinary and health-conscious voyage into the fascinating realm of Herbaceous Appetizers with "The Herbal Cookbook: Using Nature's Pharmacy in the Kitchen." These appetizers, infused with the health of natural herbs, promise to be a lovely beginning to your culinary explorations.

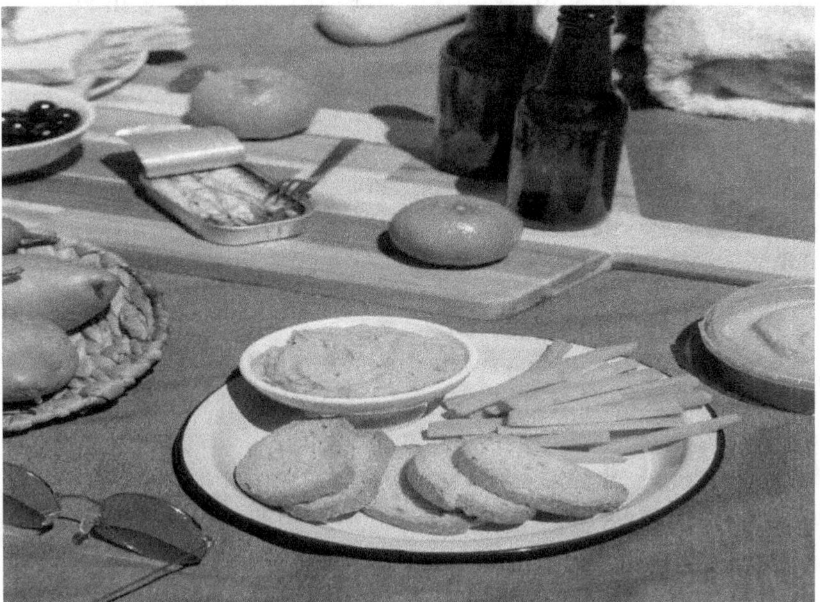

1. Bruschetta with fresh herbs: With each mouthful, the Fresh Herb Bruschetta delivers a blast of freshness thanks to a delectable combination of nature's best tastes. This appetizer honors the freshness and adaptability of herbs right from the garden and perfectly encapsulates our herbal culinary adventure. Ripe tomatoes, aromatic basil, and other carefully chosen herbs are combined in this dish, which is a symphony of flavors and colors that not only tantalizes the taste senses but also highlights the beauty of natural ingredients.

Toasting slices of artisanal bread until they turn golden brown is the first step in the preparation process. These are the canvases on which the herbaceous masterpiece is painted. A substantial amount of freshly chopped parsley, basil, and other fragrant herbs are combined with finely diced tomatoes to create a zesty and refreshing topping. With a dash of balsamic glaze and a drizzle of extra virgin olive oil, every bruschetta transforms into a wonderful burst of flavor. This recipe, which elevates a straightforward snack into a culinary experience that perfectly captures The Herbal Cookbook's philosophy, is a monument to the transforming power of herbs. Savor the simplicity and richness of herbal gastronomy by embracing the many gifts of nature's pharmacy in your kitchen with Fresh Herb Bruschetta.

2. The Rosemary Infused Hummus: is a prime example of the harmonious fusion of culinary creativity and the restorative power of nature inside the enchanted realm of herbal cuisine. This delicious dish perfectly combines flavor and nutrition while encapsulating the strong fragrance of rosemary and unveiling a host of health benefits.

In this hummus recipe, rosemary—an aromatic herb prized for its earthy scent and complex taste profile—takes center stage. With its addition, the classic spread made with chickpeas becomes an exquisite meal, enhanced by a well-balanced mix of zesty and piney notes. In addition to its exquisite flavor, rosemary has long been prized for its therapeutic qualities. With its ability to aid with digestion and provide an antioxidant boost, this plant becomes a culinary ally in our pursuit of overall health.

In addition to its delicious flavor, Rosemary Infused Hummus in "The Herbal Cookbook" is significant because it embodies the cookbook's idea of using nature's medicine in the kitchen. This recipe encourages readers to embrace the therapeutic power of herbs with every delicious mouthful by demonstrating how common herbs may improve the flavor and nutritional content of our meals. We set out on a trip where the kitchen becomes a haven for creative cooking as well as holistic well-being as we taste the Rosemary Infused Hummus.

3. Bits of cucumber and dill: Cucumber and dill combine to create a symphony of freshness that dances on the palate, making them a gourmet match made in herb heaven. This recipe, from "The Herbal Cookbook: Using Nature's Pharmacy in the Kitchen," is a delicious bite-sized dish that combines the crisp, watery texture of cucumbers with the earthy, lemony aromas of dill.
Cucumber and dill together have several health advantages in addition to being a palate-teasing combination. With its antioxidant and anti-inflammatory qualities, dill gives the meal an added nutritious boost. Cucumbers, on the other hand, add vital vitamins and water, making this appetizer a healthy option. These morsels are a tribute to the cookbook's philosophy,

showing how cooking with nature's medicine can improve meals.

The cookbook's dedication to use herbs for their taste and health benefits is embodied by Dill and Cucumber Bites, which may be enjoyed as a light snack, an appetizer at parties, or a side dish. With this herbal masterpiece that celebrates the combination of nature's best ingredients, get ready to go on a voyage of flavor and wellness.

4. Crostini with Basil Pesto: The Basil Pesto Crostini is a culinary masterwork that epitomizes nature's medicine in the kitchen when it comes to herb cuisine. The main ingredient in this delicious appetizer is a lively and fragrant basil pesto, which is made by combining the strong tastes of fresh basil, pine nuts, Parmesan cheese, garlic, and olive oil.

In addition to its divine flavor, Basil Pesto Crostini in "The Herbal Cookbook" is significant because it honors the culinary and therapeutic qualities of basil. The star of the show is basil, which has antibacterial and anti-inflammatory qualities that provide a health boost with every delicious taste. The crostini's texture, which is crunchy but yielding, makes it the ideal canvas for the rich pesto, which enhances the entire dining experience. This dish shows how a basic plant like basil can be turned into a gourmet marvel, demonstrating the cookbook's dedication to maximizing the potential of foods found in nature. Basil Pesto Crostini, from garden to kitchen, is a perfect example of how nature's medicine can be harmoniously integrated, transforming every meal into a sensory experience that is good for the body and the spirit.

5. Minty Melon Skewers: Found in the pages of "The Herbal Cookbook: Using Nature's Pharmacy in the Kitchen," minty melons serve as a refreshing tribute to the peaceful union of nature's wealth and culinary talent. These tasty kebabs perfectly blend the crunch of mixed melons with the energizing power of fresh mint, producing a mouthwatering snack that embodies herbal cuisine.

The importance of Minty Melon Skewers is found in its natural health advantages as well as their exquisite taste. Melons provide a healthy and moisturizing basis since they are high in vitamins and antioxidants. Not only does mint improve the flavor profile, but it also adds several health benefits. Because mint is known to have digestive benefits and to improve lung health, these skewers are not only a delicious food item but also a culinary creation that promotes wellbeing.

Minty Melon Skewers, a featured dish in "The Herbal Cookbook," are a perfect example of the cookbook's guiding principle, which is to highlight the fusion of healthful, natural ingredients with creative cooking. This recipe is a perfect example of how a kitchen can be made into a safe refuge for experimenting with the medicinal properties of fresh food and herbs.

6. Herbal Stuffed Mushrooms: A masterwork of culinary craftsmanship, Herbal Stuffed Mushrooms demonstrate how nature's medicine can be seamlessly incorporated into the center of the kitchen. These delicious little morsels highlight a well-balanced combination of fragrant herbs, transforming the common mushroom into a gourmet masterpiece. In addition to adding a taste explosion, the stuffing, which is made with a variety of carefully chosen herbs, has several health advantages. Herbs like cilantro and basil provide their own therapeutic qualities, and herbs like thyme, rosemary, and oregano infuse the mushrooms with a symphony of delicious flavors. These filled mushrooms are not only delicious, but they are also a nutritious powerhouse, providing a variety of vitamins, minerals, and antioxidants. Herbs and mushrooms come together to produce a meal that is not only delicious but also good for your health.

Herbal Stuffed Mushrooms are the epitome of The Herbal Cookbook—a classy appetizer or side dish that invites you to indulge in the bounty of nature. Accept this gastronomic adventure with us as we honor the union of herbs and mushrooms, transcending the commonplace and igniting a renewed sense of gratitude for the many riches that nature bestows onto our kitchens. In addition to demonstrating the adaptability of herbs, these Herbaceous Appetizers give a taste of the delectable treats found in "The Herbal Cookbook." Get ready to explore new heights with appetizers as we combine the culinary arts with nature's remedy cabinet.

CHAPTER 4

Soups and Stews With a Natural Flavor

Take a trip into a realm of cozy warmth and fragrant joy with the delightful "Soups & Stews Infused with Nature" chapter from "The Herbal Cookbook: Using Nature's Pharmacy in the Kitchen." This section honors the union of dietary supplements with the healing powers of nature's pharmacy.

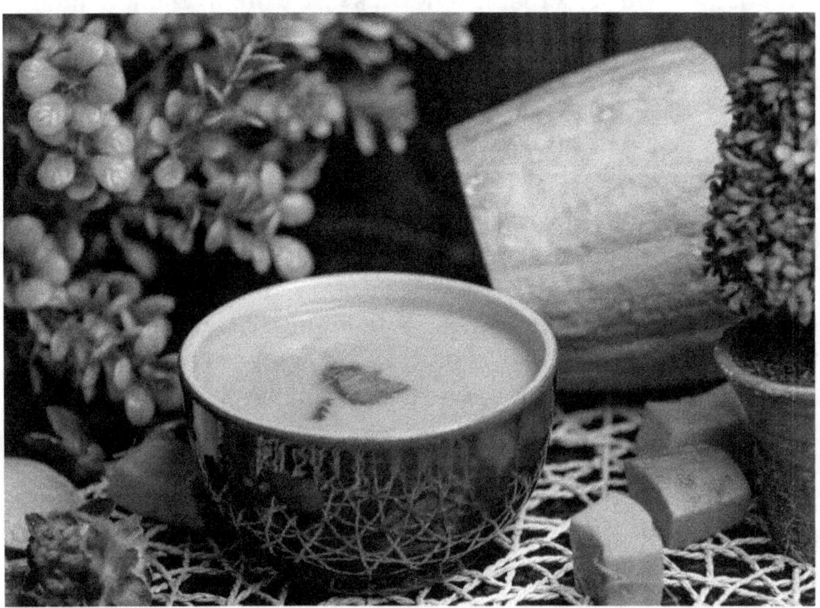

1. Comforting Bowls of Healing: Bask in the comforting embrace of "Healing Bowls of Comfort," a part of The Herbal

Cookbook where a culinary haven is created from nature's medicine. These bowls are filled to the brim with magical herbs and are designed to not only tempt your senses but also support your overall health. These bowls are a need in your herbal kitchen for the following reasons:

Holistic Wellness: Indulge in a symphony of tastes, with each component hand-selected for its unique capacity to promote holistic health.

Restorative Elixirs: Learn about bowls made to invigorate, with herbal infusions that provide a sense of rejuvenation and balance beyond simple nutrition.

Culinary Alchemy: Discover the enchanted union of nutritious foods, herbs, and spices to create concoctions that take comfort food to a whole new level of healing.

Accept Nature's Abundance: With a range of soothing herbal teas and immunity-boosting broths, these bowls use nature's medicine to improve your general well-being.

Mindful Eating: Savor each bite with awareness of the relationship between your body and mind, understanding that each component enhances not just flavor but also your overall health.

2. A Symphony of tastes: Take a culinary adventure that creates a symphony of tastes in "The Herbal Cookbook: Using Nature's Pharmacy in the Kitchen," and elevate your meals to new heights. Herbs add a pleasant flavor to food, but there are many other health benefits to incorporating them into your cuisine as well. Imagine your kitchen as a colorful garden where every herb is a distinct note in a symphony, combining to produce delectable culinary marvels.

Harness the fragrant power of herbs to unlock the potential of nature's medicine and turn ordinary meals into memorable experiences. Herbs give your food a vibrant, nuanced, and freshly made taste. They are nutritional powerhouses that provide vitamins, antioxidants, and other vital components to your food preparations. They are not simply taste enhancers. Create enticing and visually appealing meals with highlights such as "Minty Crescendo," which highlights the cooling effect of mint in sweets, or "Basil's Bold Ballet," which highlights the peppery kick of the herb. This symphony isn't limited to any one food; rather, it's a worldwide culinary passport that lets you create a variety of delectable songs in your kitchen. Taste buds will dance to the symphony of tastes composed by "The Herbal Cookbook." Savor the delight of cooking with the organic rhythms and melodies of herbs.

3. Rejuvenate Every Drink: Using Natural Medicine in the Culinary Arts. Boost your health as you learn about the healing properties of herbal drinks. Explore the world of delicious mixtures created to stimulate your senses and provide nutrition for your body.

Nature's Remedy: Take a sip of herbal infusions and feel the healing power of nature's goodness filling you up. Discover the healing power of plants, from balancing chamomile to stimulating peppermint.

Discover the beyond-taste advantages of herbal elixirs for holistic wellness. Increase digestion, fortify your immune system, and discover peace with each cup. It's a complete wellness ritual rather than just a drink.

Take a Drink and Relax: Relax with herbal teas that are meant to calm your spirit. Discover the art of relaxation in a cup with a soothing lavender mix or a stress-relieving chamomile infusion.

In " Rejuvenate Every Drink," learn how nature's pharmacy can turn common beverages into remarkable elixirs that will infuse your everyday activities with health and vigor. Accept the healing properties of herbal drinks, and let each sip be a step toward a more vibrant self.

4. Sensations of the Seasons: Welcome to "The Herbal Cookbook: Using Nature's Pharmacy in the Kitchen," an enchanting world where we explore the beautiful world of Seasonal Sensations through a culinary journey through the seasons. Take in the ever-changing tapestry of flavors, colors, and scents as we use nature's medicine to enhance your food to a whole new level.

Harvest Harmony: Learn how to create recipes that highlight the abundance of each season by experiencing the symphony of seasonal herbs dancing in perfect harmony with fresh food. Awakening of Spring: Taste buds awakened by bright plants emerging from their winter hibernation. Savor the invigorating essence of spring with everything from fiery minty treats to delicate salads laced with chives.

Summer Herb Fiesta: Savor the mouthwatering flavors of summer, when herbs like basil, rosemary, and cilantro take center stage in crisp salads, mouthwatering grilled dishes, and enticing herbal-infused drinks.

Autumn Spice Extravaganza: Our food creations transform in color alongside the changing foliage. Savor the comforting flavors of fall, such as thyme-infused comfort meals, sage-kissed soups, and dishes flavored with cinnamon.

Winter Herbal Elegance: Add a feast of herbal elegance to your winter paradise. Taste the powerful flavors of roasts seasoned with rosemary, calming teas made with chamomile, and filling stews made with the flavor of winter herbs.

Herbal Rainbow Delights: Add joy and vibrancy to your plate with herbal concoctions that span the spectrum of colors and flavors. Taste the rainbow.

The dishes in "The Herbal Cookbook"'s Seasonal Sensations are more than simply recipes; they're a celebration of nature's abundance and a tribute to the seasons' constant change, which motivates us to create culinary masterpieces enhanced with the healing power of herbs. Come experience the harmony of nature's medicine in your kitchen as we appreciate the changing seasons.

5. Herbal Remedies: Herbal Remedies for Well-Being:
Discover how to make magical recipes that can improve your health in this section of "The Herbal Cookbook: Using Nature's Pharmacy in the Kitchen." Explore the healing realm of herbal elixirs that are intended to revitalize and replenish. With the help of nature's medicine, these elixirs can improve your culinary adventure's flavor and health.
Discover the possibilities of herbal alchemy by investigating elixirs that are purposefully and intentionally made. Each dish showcases the many ways that herbs may be used outside of the typical kitchen, from soothing chamomile infusions to energizing ginger combinations. they are not your average drinks; they are elixirs of energy that let you incorporate herbal wisdom into your everyday routine.

Learn about the many benefits of these herbal elixirs, which include strengthening immune system function, easing stress, and improving digestion. Learn how to make an immune-boosting elderberry elixir or a relaxing lavender-infused mixture to help you relax at the end of the day. The act of drinking these herbal elixirs can promote overall wellbeing; the possibilities are as varied as nature itself. These herbal elixirs can help you transform your kitchen into a paradise for holistic nourishment as well as culinary delights.

Gourmet Ease: When it comes to cooking magic, "Gourmet Simplicity" is the driving concept of "The Herbal Cookbook: Using Nature's Pharmacy in the Kitchen." This area embraces the simplicity that turns everyday meals become memorable experiences, deftly weaving together a delicate tapestry of tastes gleaned from nature's own pharmacy.

Herbs are the unsung superstars in this case; their fragrant charm and nutritional value elevate any dish. Savor the beautiful simplicity of a Basil Pesto Pasta, where Parmesan, pine nuts, and fresh basil combine to create a palate-pleasing symphony of flavors. Taste the invigorating power of Minted Citrus Salad, where citrus fruits and mint leaves dance to awaken the senses. "Gourmet Simplicity" pushes the envelope by adding a sophisticated herbal flavor to food without being overly complicated. Learn how to infuse herbal oils into roasted veggies or grilled meats for a subtle yet significant effect. Allow the cookbook to lead you through the process of making a Rosemary Lemonade, which combines the citrus appeal of lemons with the earthy undertones of rosemary to create a drink that perfectly embodies elegance without sacrificing simplicity. Discover the enchantment in the little things as your kitchen becomes a herbal refuge that celebrates the marriage of the finest cuisine and nature's medicine.

CHAPTER 5

Healthy Herbal Salads & Dressings

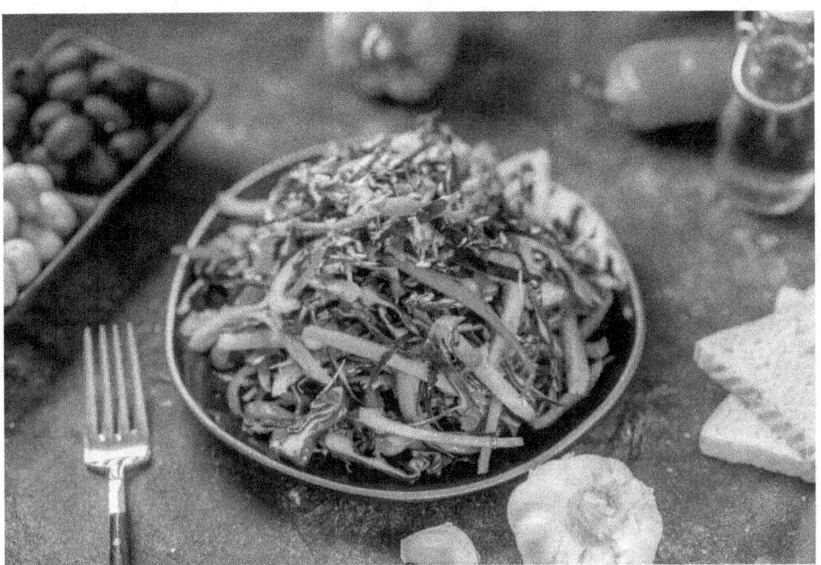

When it comes to culinary treats, salads and dressings are the stars because they provide a blank canvas for creativity and a blast of cool tastes. With 'Herbalicious Salads & Dressings,' a chapter that turns common greens into spectacular culinary masterpieces, you can embrace the culinary magic of herbs in your salads.

1. Harmony of Newness: Enter a world of freshness where scented herbs mingle with vivid greens. Every morsel is an ode to the abundance of nature, a palate-pleasing symphony.

2. Basil Bliss Dressing: This dressing, which combines olive oil and balsamic vinegar with the earthy tones of basil, will up your salad game. It's an amazing experience rather than merely a dressing.

3. Minty Citrus Delight: Our Minty Citrus Delight offers a refreshing experience in a different way. The refreshing embrace of mint combines with zesty citrus flavors to create a salad that is more than simply a meal.

4. Greens Infused with Thyme: Discover the ageless charm of thyme for your salads. Its delicate, woodsy overtones give your greens more depth and elevate a basic salad to a fine dining experience.
5. Parsley Passion Salad: Infuse your salad dish with the passion of parsley. This herb gives every taste a blast of freshness and a touch of peppery charm with its vibrant green tint.

6. Dill-icious Avocado Ensemble: Dill and avocado are a marriage made in heaven. Your taste senses will be singing as the creamy smoothness of avocado and the fragrant, slightly tart dill combine to produce a lovely duet.

7. Sage and Honey Elegance: Savor the sophistication of sage as it unites with the delectability of honey. This dressing transforms your salad into a sophisticated culinary masterpiece with its ideal ratio of salty to sweet.

8. Unleash the Magic of Rosemary in a Vinaigrette: Transform common greens into a sensory extravaganza with this simple yet elegant recipe. This dressing is a gourmet delight, not simply a condiment.

9. Lavender Lemonade Drizzle: Imagine a light floral accent being added to your salad by a lavender-infused lemonade that drizzles over it. It's a fragrant trip through lavender fields, not simply a dressing.

10. Cilantro Lime Fiesta: This zesty dressing will take your taste senses to a vibrant fiesta. On your plate, the zest of lime and the robust flavors of cilantro create a party.

11. Tarragon Tango Salad: This salad laced with tarragon will make you dance with its exquisite nuances. Its subtle anise taste gives your greens a sophisticated touch.

12. Oregano Olive Symphony: Immerse yourself with the Oregano Olive Symphony, where the richness of olives and the powerful notes of oregano blend harmoniously. It's a salad bowl party with a touch of the Mediterranean.

13. Chamomile Citrus exhilaration: Experience exhilaration with a dressing of chamomile and citrus. Bright citrus notes blend with the relaxing aroma of chamomile to create a dressing that is both exhilarating and comforting.

14. Coriander Spice Fusion: Use coriander to start a voyage of spice fusion. Your salads take on a unique twist from its warm, zesty flavor, leaving you with amazing dining experiences.

15. Herbs de Provence Elegance: In your salad, savor the timeless elegance of herbs de Provence. This classic herb combination gives your dishes a hint of French refinement.

Every mouthful in "Healthy Herbal & Dressings" is an ode to nature's medicine, with herbs taking center stage in converting your kitchen into a gourmet paradise. Elevate your salads, entice your palate, and watch as the culinary symphony of herbs materializes on your plate.

CHAPTER 6

Enjoy the Herbal Appetizers

Discover the remarkable realm of plant-based main courses as we explore the core of "The Herbal Cookbook: Using Nature's Pharmacy in the Kitchen." We set out on a quest to elevate everyday meals into spectacular culinary experiences in this area. Get ready for a delightful journey through herbs that not only improve flavor but also impart the health and nutritional advantages of nature's pharmacy into every meal.

Perfect Tomato Pasta with a Basil Infusion: Savor a pasta dish that combines the flavorful potency of tomatoes with the fragrant qualities of basil, creating a symphony of tastes. Learn how basil adds antioxidants to promote your health in addition to enhancing flavor.

Experience the enchantment of rosemary as it elevates a basic roasted chicken dish to a gourmet masterpiece in this recipe for Rosemary Roasted Chicken Bliss. Learn about the health advantages of rosemary, including better digestion and possible anti-inflammatory effects.

Garlic With Thyme Infusion Shrimp Delight: A shrimp meal that entices the senses with the interplay of thyme, lemon, and garlic will take you on a flavorful voyage. Examine the ways that thyme may enhance flavor and possibly strengthen the immune system.

Sage-Buttered Sweet Potato Gnocchi: Savor the reassuring touch of butter flavored with sage when it drizzles over these potato skins. Discover the many applications of sage in cooking and its possible function in enhancing brain wellness.

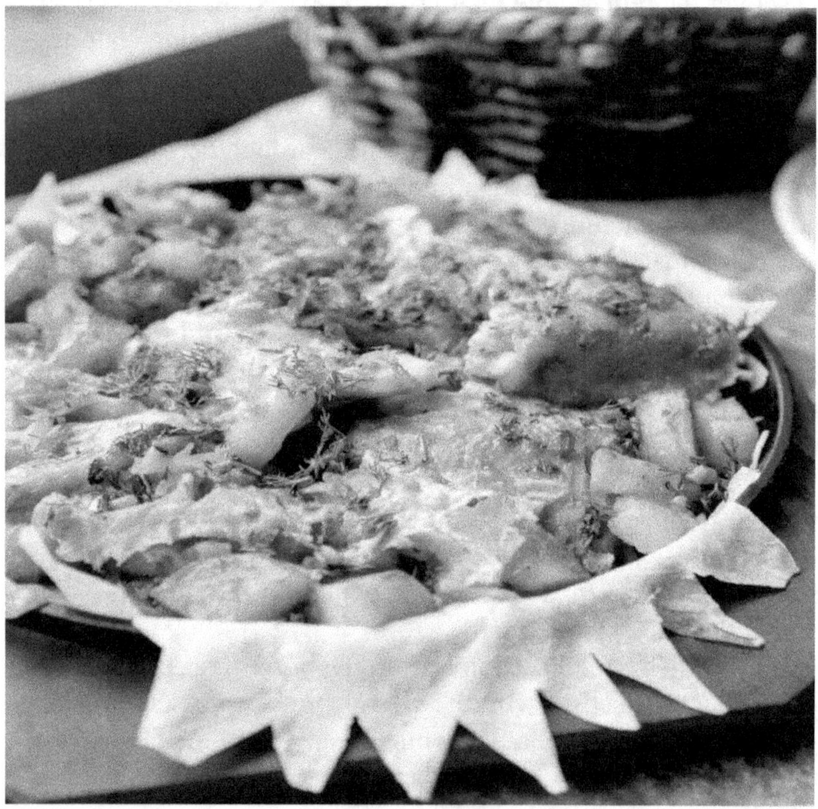

Minty Lamb Chops with Pomegranate Glaze: This meal of delicious lamb chops will wow your senses with the union of mint and pomegranate. Discover the health advantages of mint for digestion and the antioxidant power of pomegranates.

Cilantro Lime Grilled Fish Tacos: These grilled fish tacos with a hint of lime and cilantro will take your taste buds to a fiesta of sensations. Savor the crisp brightness of lime and the reviving properties of cilantro.

Dill-Lemon Salmon En Papillote: This dish, baked to perfection in parchment paper, elevates your salmon experience with a subtle paring of dill and lemon. Learn about the immune-stimulating capabilities of lemon and the possible anti-inflammatory qualities of dill.

Tofu Stir-Fry with Coriander-Crusted Tofu: Savor the vibrant fusion of coriander in a recipe that exemplifies how this herb can enhance the flavor and complexity of plant-based cuisine. Find out about the possible digestive advantages of coriander.

CHAPTER 7

Aromatic Pairings & Sides

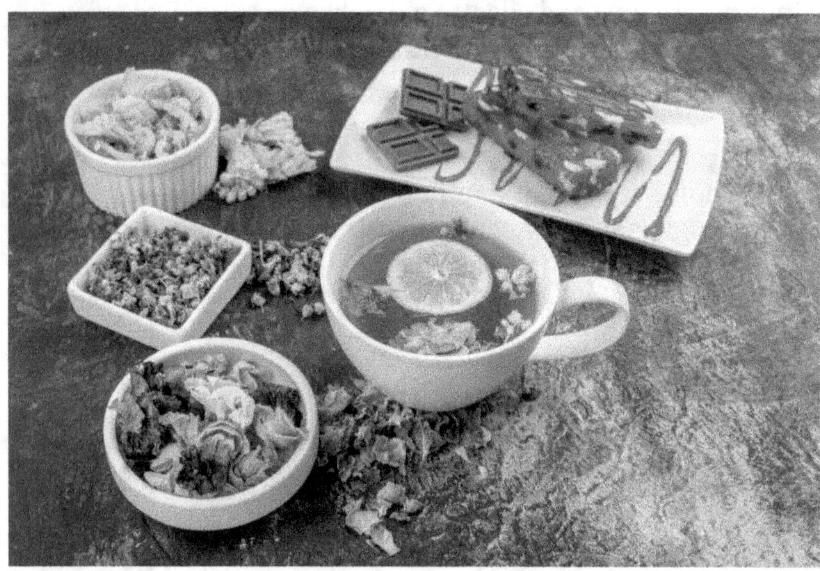

Explore the fascinating world of Aromatic Sides & Accompaniments, where you can turn everyday dishes into gourmet masterpieces thanks to nature's medicine. In this chapter of "The Herbal Cookbook," we look at how adding herbs to your side dishes improves their flavor, scent, and nutritional value, giving you a pleasurable experience with every mouthful.

1. Grains Enriched with Herbs: Transform the Typical
Find out how adding aromatic herbs can transform basic grains like rice, quinoa, and couscous into something truly remarkable.

Examples include quinoa infused with thyme, couscous flavored with parsley, and basmati rice laced with rosemary.

2. Fresh Herb Salads: A Flavorful Symphony of Colors
Discover how to use fresh herbs to make colorful, energizing salads that will entice your palate.
Examples are the watermelon salad with mint, the cilantro-lime coleslaw, and the tomato and basil salad.

3. Herbal Spreads & Butters: Give Love
Take your snacking game to the next level by adding handmade herb-infused butters to your toast or crackers.
Examples are dill-infused cream cheese, olive tapenade flavored with rosemary, and butter flavored with garlic and chives.
4. Aromatic Roasted Vegetables: Your Plate, Inspired by Nature's Palette
Roasting veggies with a blend of fragrant herbs transforms them into a visual and gustatory treat.
Examples include butternut squash cooked with sage, potatoes roasted with oregano, and carrots roasted with thyme.

5. Herbal Infusion Dips: Tasty Dipping
Discover the world of herbal dips, ideal for serving with vegetable crudités or dipping your favorite snacks.
Hummus with basil pesto, Greek yogurt dip with dill, and cilantro-lime aioli are a few examples.

6. Unique Herbal Chutneys: International Blending
Herbal chutneys, such as cilantro-mint chutney, tarragon-infused
mango chutney, and parsley-garlic chimichurri, allow you to
"tour the world through your taste buds."

7. Botanical-Infused Oils and Vinegars: The True Nature
Use herb-infused oils and vinegars to enhance your marinades
and sauces, giving your food more flavor and depth.
Examples include balsamic vinegar infused with thyme, red
wine vinegar flavored with basil, and olive oil steeped with
rosemary.

8. Herbal Spiced Gravies: A Flavorful Explosion
Use fragrant herbs to transform classic gravies and create a
palate-exploding experience.
Examples are the tarragon-infused mushroom gravy, the parsley
and lemon caper sauce, and the sage and brown butter sauce.

Discover these Aromatic Sides & Accompaniments and learn
the art of herbal infusion, bringing nature's medicine right into
your kitchen. Give each meal the opportunity to tell a tale of
taste, aroma, and the amazing possibilities that come from
giving herbs the spotlight in your cooking.

CHAPTER 8

Add Some Flavor to Your Breakfasts

Awaken to the enticing scents and bright tastes of breakfasts enriched with herbs! In this part, we'll look at some inventive methods to combine nature's pharmacy with culinary art to turn your morning meals into a herbal symphony.

1. Shine Brightly Elixirs
Discover energizing herbal teas and morning elixirs to get your day going.
An example would be a zesty spin on citrus mint infusion.

2. Super Herbal Breakfast Bowls
Find filling bowls that are bursting with herbs to give you a boost.
For instance, a bowl of Basil Berry Bliss drizzled with honey.

3. Fresh Omelets from the Garden
Garden greens and aromatic herbs will up your omelette game.
For instance: Dill and Chive Delight Omelet.

4. An Orchestra of Medicinal Pancakes

Make your pancakes into a delectable herb-infused treat.
Example: Sweet-tasting lavender-lemon pancakes.

5. Nutritious Herbal Drinks

Smoothie your way to a plant-based paradise with wholesome drinks.
For a cool change, try a Minty Green Goddess Smoothie.

6. Porridge laced with herbs

Comforting herbal porridge to warm you up in the mornings.
For instance, cinnamon sage A comforting start with Spice Porridge.

7. Herbal Delights Toast

Upgrade your toasts with toppings and spreads made of herbs.
Example: For a savory taste, try avocado toast laced with thyme.

8. Morning Baking Extravaganza

For a filling breakfast, bake some delicious treats with a hint of herbs.
Breakfast casserole with a rosemary scent, for instance.

9. Revitalizing Herbal Concoctions

Discover invigorating morning beverages and water blended with herbs.
Example: Enliven your day with Ginger Lemongrass Infused Water.

10. Morning Parfaits with Herbs - Enliven your morning with delectable parfaits made with herbs. A tasty example might be a blueberry-basil parfait.

Use the Herbal Cookbook as a guide to create mornings that are full of the goodness of the natural world. Elevate your breakfasts by adding the flavor of rich herbs and the hope of a colorful day ahead to every meal. Breakfast is a festival of flavors and a nutritious routine to appreciate the beauty of every morning, after all. It's more than simply a meal.

CHAPTER 9

Herbal Infusions & Beverages

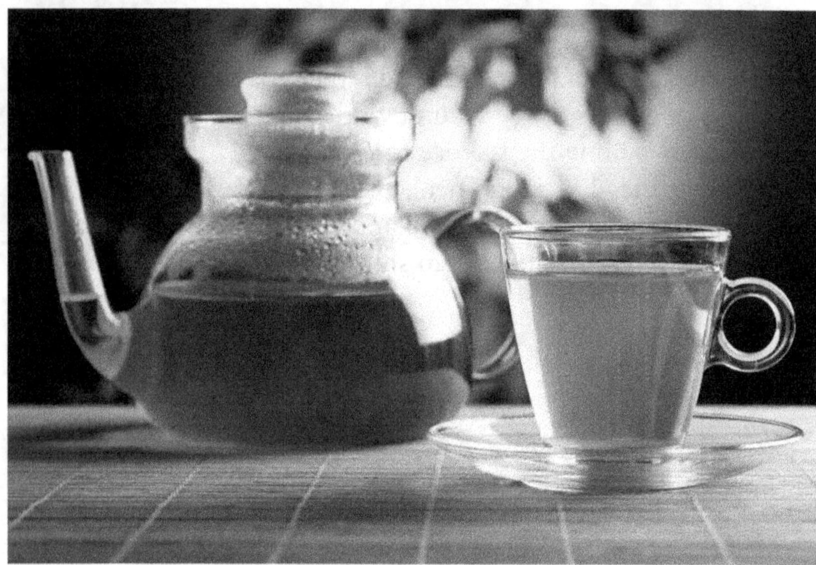

Beverages and infusions, in the enchanted realm of herbal mixtures, are a monument to the union of nature's pharmacy and the culinary arts. This chapter of "The Herbal Cookbook: Using Nature's Pharmacy in the Kitchen" explores the flavorful world of herbal beverages, offering a cool diversion and an exploration of the diverse tastes and health benefits found in nature's bounty.

1. Teas made with herbs:
In this chapter, herbal teas, with their soothing warmth and healing qualities, take center stage. The options are unlimited, ranging from the energizing peppermint tea to the soothing

chamomile infusion. Accept the calming effects of herbal concoctions, such as ginger and turmeric to strengthen immunity or lavender and lemon balm to promote relaxation. An example of a recipe might be "Energizing Hibiscus Citrus Tea," which is a refreshing blend of orange peel, mint, and hibiscus blossoms.

2. Infused Waters: In the realm of infused waters, flavor and hydration combine. Increase the amount of water you drink each day by adding infusions of herbs like cilantro, mint, and basil. A dish that combines the refreshing scent of fresh mint leaves with the sharpness of cucumber is called "Cucumber Mint Infusion," and it sounds really tasty.

3. Herbal Lemonades: By adding aromatic herbs, you may turn the traditional lemonade into a herbal treat. Take the "Rosemary Lemonade," which combines the sharpness of the lemons with the woodsy tones of rosemary to create a delightful drink that looks as good as it tastes.

4. Medicinal Tisanes: Use tisanes to delve into the therapeutic aspects of herbal drinks. Explore the realm of therapeutic infusions with recipes like "Ginger Turmeric Tisane," which combines these powerful herbs to create a beverage that has anti-inflammatory properties in addition to being really tasty.

5. Herbal Iced Teas: A refreshing take on classic tea blends, herbal iced teas are ideal for hot days. A tempting choice would be the "Berry Basil Iced Tea," which is a summertime-inspired drink that combines the aromatic freshness of basil with the sweetness of berries.

6. Calm Herbal Concoctions:
Relax with herbal tinctures that are meant to calm the spirit. Discover the soothing properties of lavender and chamomile with the "Tranquil Lavender Chamomile Elixir," a drink that helps you get into a peaceful night's sleep and serves as a bedtime ritual.

7. Herbal Concoctions:
Herbal smoothies are a great way to add the health benefits of herbs into your daily routine. Combine kale, pineapple, and cilantro in a blender and create a colorful drink called "Green Goddess Smoothie," which is full of nutrients and has a cool herbal taste.

8. Fermented Herbal Drinks: Explore the realm of fermentation with the addition of herbal flavors. Try making a "Probiotic Mint Ginger Brew," which combines the digestive powers of ginger and mint with the health advantages of fermentation.

9. Herbal Cocktails: Herbal cocktails take center stage for those looking for a sophisticated take on herbal pleasure. Make a "Basil Berry Gin Fizz" to experience a delicious fusion of elegant spirit and herbal freshness.

10. Revitalizing Herbal Elixirs: Act as natural pick-me-ups by invigorating your senses with herbal elixirs. As an illustration, consider the "Citrus Rosemary Revitalizer," a zesty blend that combines the energizing scent of rosemary with the brightness of citrus fruits.

11. Mocktails with Herbs:
Herbal mocktails, not to be outdone, provide a flavor-forward non-alcoholic substitute. For a joyful drink without the alcohol content, try the "Sparkling Mint Berry Cooler," a dazzling blend of berries, mint, and sparkling water.

12. Juices with infused herbs:
Try these herbal infusions to liven up your everyday juice regimen. One such would be the "Turmeric Pineapple Wellness Juice," a colorful concoction that combines the benefits of pineapple sweetness with turmeric powder to strengthen immunity and improve overall health.

13. Original Herbal Concoctions:
Try blending some unusual herbal mixtures and let your imagination go wild. For a unique herbal experience, create a "Lemongrass Lavender Fusion," combining the zesty notes of lemongrass with the delicate floral notes of lavender.

14. Herbal Drinks that are Seasonal:
Make your herbal drinks appropriate for the season to help you
embrace the shifting of the seasons. For fall, try making a
"Spiced Apple Sage Cider" that combines the earthiness of sage
with the warmth of spices.

15. Herbal Hydration for Health: Summarize the advantages
of herbal drinks to wrap up our investigation of them. Talk
about the moisturizing qualities of infused waters, the immune-
boosting potential of different herbal combinations, and the
antioxidant-rich nature of herbal teas.

Regarding herbal drinks and infusions, "The Herbal Cookbook"
reveals a rich tapestry of tastes, aromas, and health advantages.
Enjoy the symphony of nature's brews in your own kitchen with
the herbal delights found inside these pages, whether you're
looking for a soothing cup before bed or a revitalizing elixir to
start your day.

CHAPTER 10

Sweet Herbal Treats

With "The Herbal Cookbook: Using Nature's Pharmacy in the Kitchen," we take a wonderful tour of the world of delicious herbal confections. Through the use of colorful and fragrant ingredients from nature's garden, we bring classic desserts to a whole new flavor and nutritional level. We'll explore several types of sweet herbal sweets in this excursion, offering ideas and direction to the inexperienced cook as well as the seasoned one.

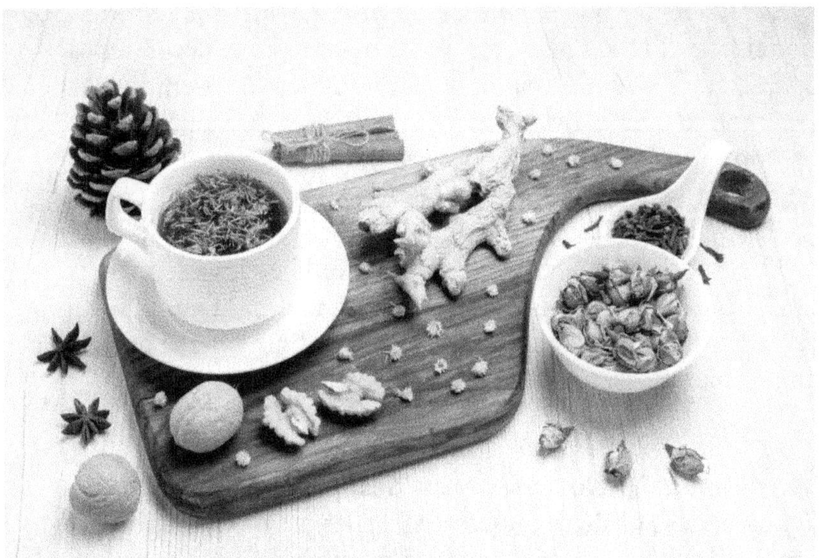

Basics of Herbal-Infused Desserts:
Let's first go over the fundamentals of adding herbs to sweets

before getting into particular recipes. Herbs can be utilized in a variety of ways, such as extracts, dried, or fresh. For example, you may steep mint in cream to make a cool ice cream, or you can infuse sugar with lavender to make a fragrant cake.

Cupcakes with lavender lemonade:

Lavender lemonade cupcakes are a prime example of the allure of herbal treats; they have the ideal balance of flowery aromas and zesty acidity. The delicate aroma of lavender-infused sugar balances the tart lemon taste of the cupcakes. This careful balancing act demonstrates how herbs may elevate a traditional dessert's overall pleasure.

Shortbread Cookies with Rosemary Honey:

These rosemary honey shortbread biscuits will convert you even if you don't think savory rosemary belongs in a sweet delicacy. The honey's sweetness and the earthy notes of rosemary combine to create a very tasty biscuit. They are a unique addition to your repertoire of herbal desserts because of their texture and scent.

Taste the pleasant world of herbal sorbets with this delightful basil berry sorbet. The richness of mixed berries is enhanced by the herbaceous tones of basil, resulting in a light and refreshing frozen delight. It's a perfect illustration of how herbs can elevate an ordinary dessert to a gourmet masterpiece.

Thyme-infused Chocolate Truffles: Savor the rich deliciousness of these chocolate truffles as you indulge your senses. The delicate earthiness of thyme balances the rich tastes of dark chocolate, giving this traditional dessert a refined edge.

Herbs can bring nuance and complexity to even the most decadent desserts, as these truffles demonstrate.

A delectable panna cotta laced with chamomile: Savor the calming effects of chamomile. The rich dessert is infused with the mildly flowery aroma of chamomile, adding a soothing touch to your post-dinner treat. This recipe shows how adding herbs to sweets may give them a more balanced flavor while also improving overall health.

Sage and Brown Butter Blondies: These blondies take a savory herb like sage and transform it into a delightful discovery. The richness of brown butter is counterbalanced by the fragrant, slightly spicy tones of sage, resulting in a chewy, delicious blondie that elevates itself above the average dessert. It's evidence of how adaptable herbs are in the kitchen.

Mint Chocolate Chip Ice Cream: Adding fresh mint leaves to the traditional mint chocolate chip ice cream elevates it. Mint leaves infuse the cream with a naturally occurring, vivid green color and a refreshing flavor that outshines manufactured substitutes. This handmade version is a great example of how herbs can bring out the flavor of a popular dessert.

Lemon Verbena and Blueberry acidic: Savor the marriage of acidic lemon flavor and juicy blueberries in this tart. The vibrant, lemony flavor of the fragrant lemon verbena perfectly balances the sweetness of the blueberries. This tart is an example of how herbs may take center stage in a dessert and elevate it to the level of a culinary masterpiece.

Cinnamon Basil Apple Crisp: The addition of cinnamon basil elevates the traditional apple crisp. The sweetness of baked apples is complemented by the warm, spicy undertones of cinnamon basil, making for a cozy and fragrant dessert. This take on a time-honored staple demonstrates how herbs can infuse familiar delicacies with creativity and complexity.

Herbal Honey Drizzled Baklava: Try this baklava with a herbal honey drizzle to discover the Mediterranean influence in herbal sweets. The sweet syrup that envelops the layers of phyllo dough and almonds provides richness when honey is infused with herbs like oregano or thyme. This treat exemplifies the adaptability of herbs in sweets from throughout the world, presenting a wonderful mix of cultures.

Sage-infused Peach Sorbet: Infuse ripe peaches with sage to create a surprising and delightful sorbet. Sage's herbal overtones bring out the richness of the peaches to create a delightfully refined and palate-cleansing ice treat. It's a perfect illustration of how herbs can take basic, in-season items and turn them into gourmet fare.

Cardamom Rosewater Rice Pudding: This rice pudding crosses ethnic barriers and takes your taste buds on an exotic voyage. This comfortable dessert combines the flowery flavor of rosewater with the warm spice of cardamom. It demonstrates how herbs can elevate a simple dish to a fragrant, far-off delight. sandwich with lemon sorbet and basil:

Try making basil lemon sorbet sandwiches to shake up your usual ice cream sandwich experience. The pleasant contrast of flavors and textures is achieved when the herbaceous sorbet is sandwiched between two lemony biscuits. This fun dish shows how herbs can liven up traditional desserts and bring in some excitement and freshness.

Chocolate Lavender Mousse: Conclude our study of sweet floral delicacies with a luscious chocolate lavender mousse. The flowery flavors of lavender softly infiltrate the rich chocolate foundation, producing a refined and delectable treat. This final dish encompasses the essence of herbal sweets — a harmonic balance of nature's tastes to produce unique and pleasurable culinary experiences.

In "The Herbal Cookbook: Using Nature's Pharmacy in the Kitchen," the chapter on sweet herbal delights unveils a world of possibilities where herbs and sweets dance together in perfect harmony. From the refreshing Basil Berry Sorbet to the luscious Chocolate Lavender Mousse, each dish displays the transformational power of herbs in the domain of sweets. Whether you're a seasoned chef or a newbie in the kitchen, these recipes inspire you to explore, create, and relish the amazing sensations that nature's pharmacy has to offer.

CHAPTER 11

Adventures in Herbal Baking

Herbal Baking Adventures: Using Nature's Bounty to Enhance
Sweet and Savory Delights
Herbal baking is one of the most exciting culinary adventures
there is, fusing the skill of baking with the fragrant marvels of
nature. We go on a voyage into the realm of Herbal Baking
Adventures in this portion of "The Herbal Cookbook: Using
Nature's Pharmacy in the Kitchen," learning how the infusion of
herbs can turn ordinary baked items into gourmet wonders.

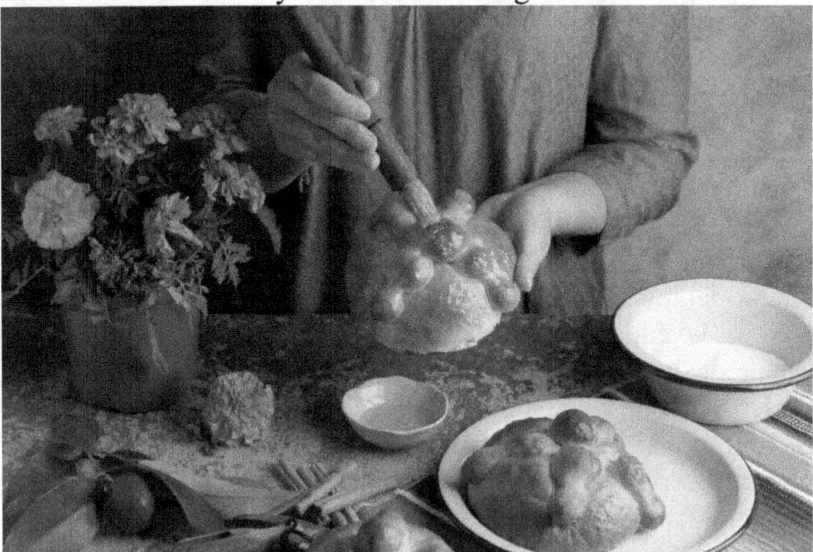

1. Basil-infused Lemon Pound Cake: Described as moist and
delicate, this pound cake combines the sweet, earthy aromas of

basil with the zesty freshness of lemons. A traditional dessert gets an unexpected twist from this unusual mix, making it a delightful and refreshing treat.
Baking Tip: To ensure that the flavor is distributed evenly, finely cut fresh basil leaves and add them to the batter. The zesty sharpness of lemon zest contrasts well with the fragrant flavor of basil.

2. Rosemary Olive Oil Focaccia: This tasty focaccia, enhanced with the aromatic flavor of rosemary, will elevate your bread-making abilities to new heights. The richness of the olive oil and the herbaceous scent of the rosemary combine to create a chewy, delicious bread that is ideal for sharing.
Baking Tip: Warm the olive oil and rosemary together over low heat so that the oil absorbs the aroma of the herb. For an added flavor boost, liberally brush the focaccia with the infused oil before baking.

3. Lavender Honey Butter Cookies: Described as taking the traditional butter cookie to a whole new level, the subtle floral notes of lavender and the sweetness of honey combine to create a delicious treat. These cookies are a delicious treat for the senses in addition to being aesthetically pleasing.
Baking Tip: Use a little amount of culinary lavender buds to prevent overpowering the cookies' flavor with soap. Melt butter and add lavender-infused honey to make a rich, fragrant cookie dough.

4. Thyme and Parmesan Scones: Described as follows: Infuse the earthy, woodsy flavor of thyme with the sharp taste of Parmesan cheese to elevate the basic scone to a delicious pleasure. These scones go well with soups and salads or as a side dish for breakfast.

Baking Tip: Grate some Parmesan cheese and finely cut some fresh thyme right into the scone batter. The scones are filled with the aromatic flavor of thyme, which makes them a savory pastry that goes well with a variety of foods.

5. Chai Spiced Cinnamon Rolls: Description: Infuse the dough with cardamom, cinnamon, and cloves to give the traditional cinnamon roll a warm and fragrant touch. The outcome is a tasty pastry that takes you back to a warm tea party and is comfortable and savory.

Baking Tip: Steep a chai tea bag in warm milk before adding it to the dough, or make your own chai spice mix using ground spices. The sweet and luscious cinnamon filling is made more nuanced by the fragrant spices.

6. Mint Chocolate Chip Muffins: Synopsis: In every mouthful, these chocolate chip muffins will revive your palette with their delicious mint flavor. These muffins are a popular for dessert or as a sweet snack because of the lovely contrast created by the mix of rich chocolate and refreshing mint.

Baking Tip: To infuse the muffin batter with mint flavor, finely cut fresh mint leaves or use mint essence. Add chocolate chips to balance the herbal undertones with a sweet explosion.

7. Sage and Walnut Biscuits: This recipe highlights the savory aspect of herbal baking by combining sage with crisp walnuts to create biscuits that are full of flavor. Because of their versatility, these biscuits may be eaten on their own or served with stews and soups.

Baking tip: To make sage-infused butter, melt butter with fresh sage leaves; sift butter to get rid of the leaves before mixing it into the dough for the biscuits. The end product is a buttery cookie with a little hint of herb flavor.

8. Chamomile-infused Shortbread biscuits:

Summary: Savor the subtle, soothing taste of chamomile with these soft, chewy shortbread biscuits. The traditional buttery richness of shortbread is given a distinctive twist by the flowery flavors of chamomile.
Baking Tip: Pulverize the dried chamomile flowers to a fine powder and include them into the dough for the shortbread. The cookies and a cup of herbal tea make a taste combination that goes well together.

9. Cheddar and Dill Cornbread:

Description: Infuse a traditional cornbread recipe with the savory richness of cheddar cheese and the sharp, herbaceous taste of dill. This herb-infused version of cornbread goes perfectly with thick soups and chili.

Baking Tip: For a uniform distribution of flavors, finely cut fresh dill and shred cheddar cheese into the cornbread batter. Cheese and herbs combine to make a flavorful and filling side dish.

10. Lemon Verbena-infused Blueberry Muffins:

Synopsis: Infuse the traditional blueberry muffin with the zesty, vibrant flavor of lemon verbena. These muffins have a light herbal undertone and are bursting with luscious blueberries. Last but not least, "The Herbal Cookbook"'s Herbal Baking Adventures section encourages readers to investigate the relationship between herbs and baked goods. Every dish demonstrates how the use of herbs lifts the flavors and creates a sensory-pleasing symphony of flavors and scents. These herbal baking recipes, which range from sweet to savory, show off the ingenuity and adaptability that can be achieved in the kitchen when nature's medicine and baking art collide. Cheers to your baking!

CHAPTER 12

Herbal Sauces & Condiments

The hidden heroes of the kitchen are the sauces and condiments, which elevate simple meals to outstanding gourmet creations. We explore the world of herbal sauces and condiments in "The Herbal Cookbook: Using Nature's Pharmacy in the Kitchen," where we learn how the abundance of natural herbs can enhance flavors and give each mouthful more complexity and subtlety.

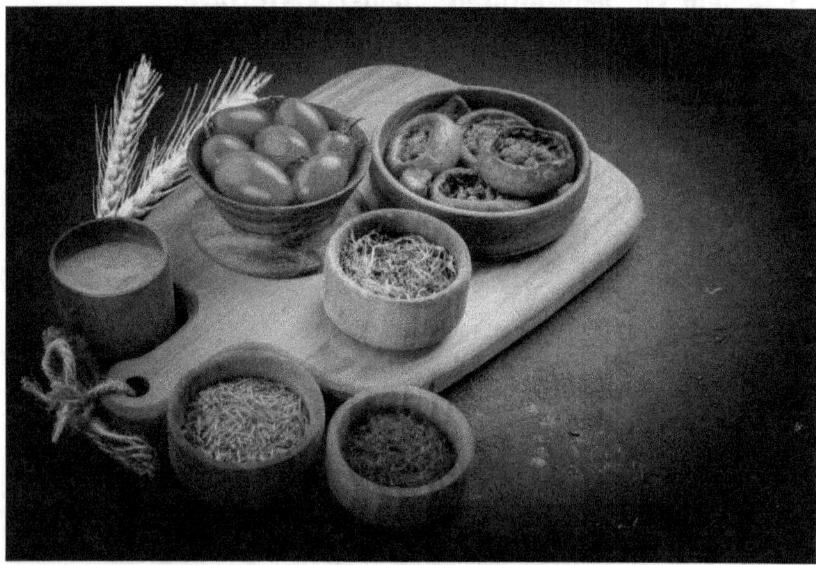

1. Pesto di Basilico: A Verdant Symphony of Tastes
This traditional pesto puts the basil, which is frequently connected to Italian cooking, front and center. This versatile herbal condiment is a blend of fresh basil leaves, garlic, pine

nuts, Parmesan cheese, and olive oil. Use it as a marinade for grilled vegetables or as a drizzle over pasta or bruschetta.

2. Mint Yogurt Sauce: A Refreshing Friend
This cool sauce mixes the pleasant taste of mint with the coolness of yogurt. Minty Yogurt Sauce is perfect as a dip for crisp vegetables or as a partner for grilled meats. It brings a refreshing blast of flavor to any cuisine.

3. Olive oil infused with rosemary: liquid gold with a hint of fragrance
Infuse your olive oil with rosemary to create a delicious elixir. This flavorful oil works well as a marinade for baked potatoes, a dip for crusty bread, or a drizzle over salads. The fragrance of rosemary gives your dishes a somewhat earthy flavor.

4. Cilantro-Lime Dressing: A Vibrant Herbal Infusion
A zesty dressing that may enhance any salad is created when you blend the zest of lime with the bright freshness of cilantro. This herb mixture also works well as a zesty spring roll dip or marinade for fish.

5. Herbal Twist on Creamy Indulgence with Dill and Mustard Aioli
Improve your aioli game by adding the unique tastes of mustard and dill. This rich, creamy treat is great as an accompaniment to

grilled chicken or as a spread over sandwiches or sweet potato fries.

6. Tarragon Shallot Vinaigrette: An Elegant French Infusion
This elegant vinaigrette will take your taste senses to France. A sauce of shallots and tarragon goes well with grilled seafood, roasted vegetables, and salads. Its faintly anise-like taste lends sophistication to your cooking projects.

7. Sage Brown Butter: A Magical Cooking Method
Watch as sage leaves dance in brown butter, a demonstration of culinary alchemy. This creamy, nutty sauce goes well with ravioli, gnocchi, or just poured over roasted veggies. Sage's herbal undertones give this straightforward yet opulent recipe depth.

8. Butter with Compound Lemon and Hazelnuts: A Vibrant Luxuriance
Serve with a dab of Chive and Lemon Compound Butter to elevate your eating experience. This buttery recipe is perfect for adding a burst of citrusy freshness to grilled meat, shellfish, or hot pasta. It also enhances the overall taste profile.

9. Honey Infused with Thyme: A Delightful Herbal Accent
When you blend the earthy tones of thyme with the sweetness of honey, you get a condiment that works well in a variety of culinary contexts. Pour thyme-infused over Use honey as a

coating on roasted meats, over cheeses, or to add a herbal edge to drinks.

10. Chimichurri with Parsley: Bright Green Delight

Argentina is the source of the colorful sauce known as chimichurri, which goes well with grilled meats. Garlic, vinegar, olive oil, and the bright flavor of parsley are all part of our variation. To bring out the vibrant green flavor of grilled steaks, try it as a marinade, dipping sauce, or topping.

11. Lavender-Fused Syrup: A Botanical Concoction

Explore the realm of elegant flowers with Lavender-infused Syrup. Perfect for adding a delicate floral note to your creations, this syrup may be used to sweeten drinks, drizzled over sweets, or mixed into inventive cocktails.

12. Oregano Tomato Sauce: A Symphony of the Mediterranean

Make a hearty tomato sauce that exudes oregano's strong scent. The Mediterranean warmth of the Oregano Tomato Sauce is perfect for pasta, pizza, or as a dipping sauce for bread.

13. A Herbal Fiesta with Coriander Lime Salsa

Turn up the heat with this colorful herbal salsa made with lime, coriander leaves, and a touch of spiciness. This salsa adds a festive flavor to any meal, whether it is served as a topping for nachos, tacos, or grilled meats.

14. Lemon Basil Mayonnaise: Creaminess with Citrus Flavor Use Lemon Basil Mayonnaise to make your sandwiches and burgers even better. The fragrant basil and zesty lemon mix to make a creamy spread that gives your favorite foods a taste boost.

15. Bay Leaf Reduction: The Key to Uncomplicated Living Simplicity is essential sometimes. A Bay Leaf Reduction is a thick and delicious reduction made by boiling bay leaves in balsamic vinegar. Use it to provide a distinctive taste to drinks or as a coating for meats or a drizzle over roasted vegetables.

These herbal sauces and condiments from "The Herbal Cookbook" are examples of culinary innovation at its most inventive. They encourage you to explore, try new things, and enjoy the amazing depth of tastes that herbs provide to your cooking by utilizing the power of nature's medicine.

CHAPTER 13

Sensations of Herbal Snacks

In the world of food exploration, snacks are frequently enjoyed as tasty breaks between meals, providing satisfying tastes and bursts of flavor. With the help of "The Herbal Cookbook: Using Nature's Pharmacy in the Kitchen," we set out to infuse common snacks with the essence and strength of nature's pharmacy, turning them into Herbal Snack Sensations.

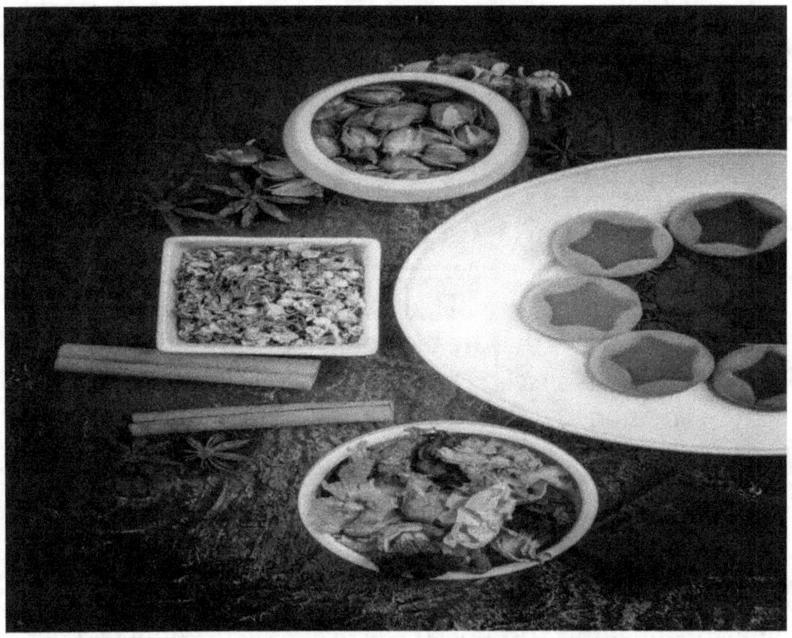

1. Delightful Herb-Infused Popcorn

Our journey into the world of herbal snacking begins with the Herb-Infused Popcorn Delight. Popcorn is a flavorful, easy-to-make snack that can inspire creative use of herbs. Think about drizzling melted butter infused with rosemary over freshly popped corn, garnished with grated Parmesan and a dash of thyme. This combination gives your snacking experience a distinct herbal scent in addition to tantalizing your taste buds.

2. Crostini with Olive Tapenade and Basil Pesto

Add some zesty flavors of olive tapenade and basil pesto to your standard crostini. The pungent basil, when mixed with pine nuts and garlic, makes a pesto that turns a plain slice of bread into a little burst of herbal bliss. For a savory twist that complements it, place a dollop of olive tapenade on top.

3. Roasted Nuts with Lavender Honey

Try the Roasted Nuts with Lavender Honey to up your nut game. This snack strikes a perfect balance between sweet, nutty, and floral notes thanks to a blend of perfectly roasted almonds, walnuts, and cashews that are then drizzled with honey infused with lavender. This snack is a visual, olfactory, and gustatory delight in addition to being delicious.

4. Kale Chips with Sea Salt and Rosemary

The best kale chips with sea salt and rosemary for guilt-free snacking are these ones. Crunchy and savory sea salt is combined with perfectly cooked kale leaves and a light drizzle of rosemary-infused olive oil. These chips provide a tasty substitute without sacrificing nutrition.

5. Vegetable Sticks with Dill and Chive Yogurt Dip

Serve a cool dill and chives yogurt dip with a variety of vibrant vegetable sticks to up your snack game. Tangy yogurt flavored with dill and chives makes a creamy, herbaceous dip that elevates common vegetables to a delightful and nourishing snack.

6. Edamame Cilantro-Lime

Cilantro Lime Edamame is a zesty way to dress up edamame. This snack is loaded with protein and bursting with flavors of citrus and herbs. It is made from steamed soybeans combined with a colorful mixture of cilantro, lime zest, and a dash of chili powder.

7. Bliss Balls of Chocolate Mint

Mint Chocolate Bliss Balls, where the indulgence of chocolate and the refreshing taste of mint, will satisfy your sweet tooth. Dates, almonds, and cocoa powder combined with a hint of fresh mint make for a delicious and guilt-free snack.

8. Potato Wedges with Sage and Parmesan

Sage's earthy flavor and Parmesan's richness elevate straightforward potato wedges to a sophisticated level. Perfectly baked to a golden brown, these wedges offer a flavorful snack with a hint of herbs, making them a hit for both parties and solitary enjoyment.

9. Shortbread Cookies with Lemon and Thyme
Thyme and Lemon Shortbread Cookies are a refreshing take on the traditional sweet cookie. A sophisticated yet comforting cookie is made when buttery shortbread is combined with the zesty zing of lemon zest and the delicate aroma of thyme.

10. A fruit salad infused with chamomile
Try a fruit salad with chamomile to revive your taste buds. A blend of seasonal fruits dipped in a mild chamomile syrup gives the traditional fruit salad a soothing and flowery touch, making it an ideal light snack for any time of day.

11. Energy Bites with Ginger Turmeric
With the potent anti-inflammatory qualities of ginger and turmeric combined with the energy-enhancing effects of nuts and dried fruits, Ginger Turmeric Energy Bites are a great way to fuel your body. These nibbles are a quick and easy on-the-go option for hectic days, in addition to being a nutritious snack.

12. Sorbet with Basil Lemonade
Basil Lemonade Sorbet transforms a refreshing beverage into a delightful frozen treat. A palate-cleansing, herbaceous sorbet that is visually pleasing and delicious is created when perfectly frozen basil-infused lemonade is combined.

13. Dark chocolate truffles with a hint of peppermint tea

Savor the rich, decadent flavor of dark chocolate truffles infused with peppermint tea. An excellent after-dinner snack, dark chocolate and peppermint tea leaves marry to create a luxurious treat that combines the cooling effect of peppermint with the boldness of chocolate.

14. Trail Mix with Herbal Infusion

Give the traditional trail mix a herbal twist to bring it back to life. Snacking has never tasted better thanks to a combination of roasted nuts, seeds, and dried fruits along with your favorite herbs like oregano, thyme, and rosemary. Each handful delivers a distinct taste explosion.

15. Pita Chips and Lemon Basil Hummus

Finish off our Herbal Snack Sensations adventure with a homemade pita chip and lemon basil hummus. With its final burst of herbal delight, the combination of crispy pita chips and creamy chickpea hummus infused with the zesty flavors of lemon and basil will have your taste buds aching for more.

Featured in "The Herbal Cookbook," these Herbal Snack Sensations redefine snacking and demonstrate the creativity and adaptability of adding herbs to regular dishes. Each recipe, which ranges from savory to sweet, takes you on a flavorful journey and demonstrates that nature's pharmacy is not only delicious but also medicinal.

CHAPTER 14

Herbal Comfort Foods

In the cozy embrace of herbal tastes, we go on a trip to explore the delightful universe of Herbal Comfort Foods. This chapter of "The Herbal Cookbook: Using Nature's Pharmacy in the Kitchen" enables you to taste the calming essence of culinary creations that provide a sense of well-being and nostalgia. We'll dig into a range of cuisines where herbs play a starring role, enriching the familiar and changing the ordinary into remarkable comfort.

1. Herbal Infused Macaroni and Cheese: Comfort food generally begins with a classic, and what's more classic than macaroni and cheese? Elevate this classic meal by infusing the creamy sauce with fresh thyme or rosemary. The herbs offer a delicate earthiness that matches the richness of the cheese, producing a warm bowl of reminiscence with a herbal twist.

2. Sage and Garlic Mashed Potatoes: Mashed potatoes, a mainstay of comfort, take on a new level with the addition of sage and garlic. The fragrant sage lends a sense of warmth, while garlic offers depth. Together, they turn a basic side into a soothing masterpiece, great for any occasion.

3. Herbal Chicken and Dumplings: Imagine a pot of sizzling chicken and dumplings with the extra charm of thyme and parsley. The herbs permeate the broth, imparting a pleasant scent that pervades the kitchen. Each mouthful becomes a trip through familiar flavors heightened by the power of herbs.

4. Rosemary-Infused Beef Stew: A hearty beef stew is a typical comfort dish, and when you throw rosemary into the mix, the outcome is remarkable. The aromatic herb enriches the flavorful broth, giving each bite a warm and fulfilling experience. This recipe is a tribute to the wonderful combination of herbs and comfort.

5. Herbal Lentil Soup: Lentil soup, a healthy staple, takes on a new level with the addition of cumin, coriander, and turmeric. This herbal infusion not only enriches the flavor but also delivers a multitude of health advantages. It's a bowl of comfort that not only warms the spirit but also boosts well-being.

6. Basil Pesto Pasta with Sun-Dried Tomatoes: Transport yourself to Italy with a comfortable dish of pasta decorated with a colorful basil pesto. The herbaceous strength of fresh basil mixed with the sweetness of sun-dried tomatoes produces a symphony of tastes that transforms a basic spaghetti dish into a cozy culinary masterpiece.

7. Chamomile and Honey Glazed Carrots: Side dishes deserve their place in the comfort limelight, and glazed carrots flavored with chamomile and honey are no exception. The soft floral notes of chamomile match the sweetness of honey, turning a modest vegetable into a side dish that offers joy and warmth to the table.

8. Lemon Verbena Rice Pudding: End your comfort feast on a sweet note with lemon verbena-infused rice pudding. The zesty scent of lemon verbena provides a pleasant twist to the creamy dessert, making it a comfortable finish to any meal. It's a great way to appreciate the sweet side of herbal comfort.

As we traverse the domain of Herbal Comfort Foods, we realize that herbs have the extraordinary capacity to lift familiar foods to new heights of delight. The union of culinary history with herbal creativity brings forth a selection of soothing dishes that not only warm the body but also nurture the spirit. In "The Herbal Cookbook," these foods serve as a tribute to the belief that nature's medicine has the potential to change the ordinary into the exceptional, one comfortable mouthful at a time.

www.ingramcontent.com/pod-product-compliance
Lightning Source LLC
Chambersburg PA
CBHW050847260726
48660CB00006B/2483